$1
8/12

Desk jobs can be hard on the body. Working at a computer can cause headaches, back pain and even mood swings. But now you can learn how to maintain well-being and counteract stress—all it takes is ten seconds to one minute—by using OFFICE YOGA.

The section called "Reduce Pain" deals with eliminating aches in the back, neck and wrists. There are sections called "Improve Efficiency" and "Increase Productivity" with tips on bettering the digestion, reducing eye-strain, staying flexible, and thinking more clearly. There is an extensive "Symptom Chart." You can look up specific targets—neck, for example—and learn which exercises to go to for relief.

Although based on traditional yoga, you don't need to be a swami to do OFFICE YOGA. In fact, the exercises are easy and pleasant and you won't even need to leave your desk or change into exercise gear.

"If you spend more than two or three hours at a desk each day you need OFFICE YOGA. Clearly written and thoroughly illustrated, OFFICE YOGA is a treasure for anyone who works at a desk."

—Wil Welsh, editor Kauai Magazine, Hawaii

"If you experience any kind of pain at home, at the office or during travel, OFFICE YOGA is the companion you will be glad you took along. Its small size is convenient to a pocket or purse. The book arrived as I was about to leave for Munich. I threw it into my bag and used it just 14 hours later at the Auberstrasser Hotel. I checked the 'Symptom Chart' for neck pain and did the exercise in two minutes—and the pain was instantly gone. Several weeks later at home, the 'Telecom Twist' exercise minimized my lower back pain. You will be glad to have a copy of OFFICE YOGA when pain or stress strikes."

—R. Joseph Jalbert, Rome, New York

"Diana Fairechild, author of JET SMARTER and NONI, has done it again: provided another concise, witty, informed, helpful guide to better health and performance. This book is going to be my friend."

—Lynn Lawson, editor Canary News, Illinois

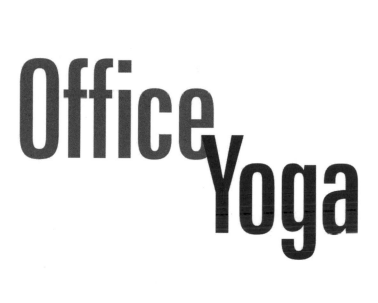

Office Yoga

by

Diana Fairechild

Copyright / Disclaimer

Office Yoga

Publisher:	**Flyana Rhyme Publishing**
Tel/Fax:	**808 828-1919**
WWW:	**www.flyana.com**
E-mail:	**diana@flyana.com**

PO Box 248, Anahola, Hawaii 96703-USA

The sole intent of the author and publisher is to offer information of a general nature. Should you choose to use this information, you are prescribing for yourself. The author and publisher assume no responsibility.

ISBN: 1-892997-40-1
LC: 00-190190
Kauai, Hawaii

Also by Diana Fairechild

JET SMARTER: The Air Traveler's Rx

The cabin of a commercial jet is one of the most sickening environments in the world. JET SMARTER offers an array of positive responses to the problem, changes in policies by the industry and also personal acts—defensive flying—that turn readers into smart flyers.

> "The perfect gift for anyone who flies and a useful tool for business travelers." General Electric Corporate Newsletter
>
> "Take the advice of Diana Fairechild."—Smart Money

NONI: Aspirin of the Ancients

The fruit of the noni tree is a rememdy used traditionally for cancer, diabetes, high blood pressure, arthritis, infertility, hair loss, poisoning, asthma, and depression. Diana took noni to detoxify from pesticide poisoning. In NONI she shares the lore and the lure of this ancient plant and its wondrous healing properties.

> "Fairechild is an authentic visionary and a gifted writer, and her latest book is a wonderful example of the healing spirit she brings to all her work."—Jonathan Krisch, Book Reviewer, Los Angeles

www.flyana.com
"Healthy Flying with Diana Fairechild"

Safe, efficient, healthy flying information on the Web

> "Fairechild advises travelers of their rights."—TIME Magazine
>
> "One of twelve most creative Web sites."—The New York Times

5

Dedication

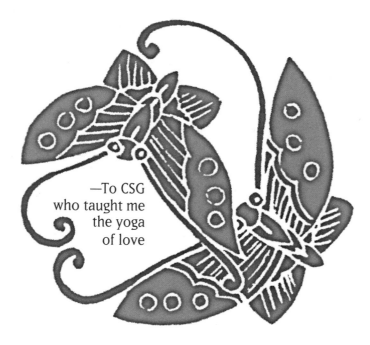

—To CSG
who taught me
the yoga
of love

Contents

Improve Efficiency

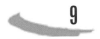

Increase Productivity.................................114

End Matter

Acknowledgments

OFFICE YOGA solidified as a system for computer health as I was completing my third book, JET SMARTER. I was under a lot of pressure because JET SMART, my first book, sold out and there were back orders. The film for JET SMART had been lost at the printer, the disks were in Mac format, and I was on a PC. When I looked at recreating a seven-year-old book, I decided I really wanted to revise it to the point of putting out a new book. For many months, I sat at my computer as much as I could, taking quick yoga breaks throughout the day—adapting traditional yoga to my computer work station.

Some of the yoga exercises that I found most useful originated as "monk yoga"—Chinese monks using yoga to keep themselves fit while sitting for long periods in meditation. When I discovered "monk yoga" I could immediately see the similarity to sitting at a computer all day, so I adapted these exercises and distilled four of them for this OFFICE YOGA series. "Cheerleader," "Rocky," "Bow and Arrow," and "Thumbs Down" are originally from the Chinese *Pal Dan Gum* monk yoga series.

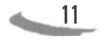

The rest of the OFFICE YOGA exercises originated in India where had I made over fifty trips during the 21 years I was an international flight attendant. During my flying years, I dropped in on classes all over the world. So, dozens of yoga teachers have influenced my own practice and thus influenced this book. I extend heartfelt thanks to all these teachers, though their names have faded from my conscious mind.

Additionally, I would like to thank four yoga teachers for directly contributing to this project: (1) Jere Graham who helped me develop some of the Indian exercises; (2) Donna Genuth who assisted me to go deeper in my own practice during the time I was writing this book; and (3) two Iyengar Yoga teachers, Brigitta Walton and Sally Cote, who reviewed the manuscript and suggested vital, subtle edits.

For the OFFICE YOGA illustrations, I extend heartfelt thanks to three people: my neighbor Ohana, who took photographs of me in the exercises, April Courture who made pencil sketches from these photos, and Chris Altemeier who skillfully and imaginatively computer-enhanced these sketches.

In a couple of the poses, I wanted the drawings to have bare feet, but Chris' computer program insisted that all the figures had to be dressed with shoes—or totally nude if we wanted bare feet. We decided to include two nudes, honoring all those who work at home.

I would also like to thank Chris Altemeier for creating the OFFICE YOGA cover, for choosing the fonts, and for technical support throughout this project.

Sincere appreciation to Weatherhill Publishing for permission to use Koyoshi Kawamoto's traditional drawings from *Elements of Japanese Design.* These Japanese family crests were first scanned, then digitally-enhanced before placing them throughout OFFICE YOGA as symbols of meditative thought. Many people have asked me what these crests were originally for. The Weatherhill book has all this information.

Thanks to Chuck and Nan Tipple for their technical support and also for taking my photo for this edition at their home overlooking the Pacific Ocean.

Appreciation to my dear yoga friend Jacqueline Levy for her savvy organizational input with this material. Thanks to Nina Andersen, Ann Ferguson, Alan Lessler, and Esther Manning for reading the manuscript at different stages and for suggesting edits.

Special appreciation is also extended to George Ewing, M.D., specialist in environmental medicine, for his inspiration.

Many thanks to Rich Lafond, Dave Sandford, and Roger Silber for insightful and essential editorial assistance and to Roger for preparing my photo for the cover and helping with my mission in many wondrous ways.

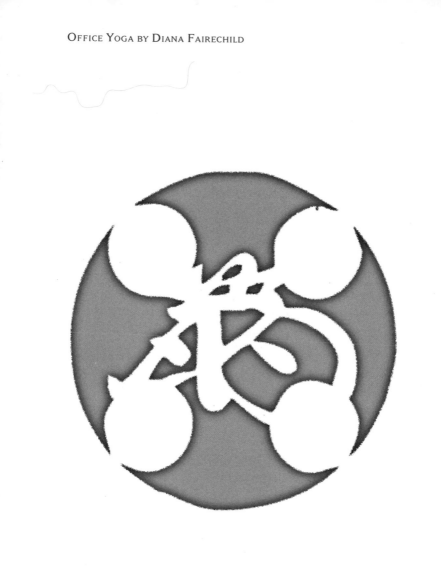

Introduction

As a writer, I have had every opportunity to experience all the bodily pains associated with sitting at a desk—headache; swollen wrists; neck, back and shoulder pains; and fuzzy thinking.

As a writer about air travel, I see my own health maintenance as similar to the way airplanes fly. It's all about self-correction. On commercial jets, for example, the pilots have to continually correct for previously unknown environmental factors such as wind, rain, and air pockets. So, in flight, they perform a series of assessments and changes to the aircraft's course, i.e., they "fly on a heading," then they check it and adjust, fly some more, check and adjust, etc.

Additionally, course changes may be initiated by controllers on the ground when they need to sequence the plane with other aircraft. The flight also has to compensate for the mechanics of the aircraft itself, such as a slight misalignment in the steering mechanism, which can vary in airplanes as it does in automobiles.

 15

In any event, no pilot expects a flight to progress without having to adjust for the many deviations from what is planned beforehand on the ground. Pilots expect adjustments to be ongoing throughout every flight.

Similarly, for our bodies to function optimally, we need to make a continuous series of adjustments in our behavior. Self-correction is an important key to well-being. Self-correction is a synonym for "yoga"—in my book. (Yoga goes much deeper, too.)

Adjustments can be made for us by physicians, chiropractors, massage therapists, acupunturists, and other health practitioners.

However, if you can self-correct on your own or work with the help of a healer, you can usually catch misalignments before they cause you downtime or long-term harm.

You can prevent the tightness and misalignments caused by office tasking with these OFFICE YOGA exercises and this, of course, will make you more effective at work. Here are two approaches. 1) Use the OFFICE YOGA exercises to relieve acute pain by referring to the "Symptom Chart" (p.36). 2) Apply the exercises as a defensive measure to help build up your balance, strength, flexibility and peace.

16

Either way, OFFICE YOGA need not take up a lot of time. Since the exercises can be performed in normal business attire right at your desk, I advice you to simply fit them in when you have a moment to spare. For example, while you wait for a page to load on the Internet, do one "Telecom Twist" (p.103) on each side. And after you return to your desk from an errand, do an "Alarm Neutralizer" (p.87). All you need is 10 seconds to one minute here and there.

These at-your-desk, user-friendly exercises are a direct application of the most advanced information about flexibility as it relates to the rigid routines of the contemporary workplace. Little by little, the exercises will also give you an experience of the extraordinary healing powers of yoga—first-hand knowledge of the body/mind/spirit connections that yoga is so famous for. I don't mean this in a religious sense, but more in terms of the self-knowledge that comes to us naturally when we pay attention. So, closely observe all sensations the way pilots watch the dials on the aircraft's instrument panel!

To start with, listen to the internal chatter of your mind—you may even hear voices. In my case, these voices are more audible to me while doing yoga than at any other time—commenting on all the different sensations which occur while I stretch.

For many people OFFICE YOGA is a resource for creativity. During the exercises answers readily bubble up—with insights relevant to personal and business problems.

Additionally, in the everyday bustle we think of as "keeping busy," fears, long forgotten, can surface—but this happens within one's control, making it possible to re-prioritize these past traumatic events. For example, while doing an OFFICE YOGA exercise, you may recall a past stressful event. I think of these memories as part of my emotional video library—during yoga my subconscious may choose a memory for me to watch, so I watch it. But I am in yoga, so I can remain detached. When I complete the exercise, I simply put the "video" away, not needing to watch it over and over. I find that I am truly bored with these old stories and they seem irrelevant when compared to the deep relaxation and other perks, such as insights, which are also available to me while doing yoga.

Practicing OFFICE YOGA is more about allowing insights and awarenesses to flow into consciousness—as water easily flows into new channels—rather than expecting results and setting specific goals. Nevertheless, with each exercise you will find a suggested goal standard, i.e. "Time to Achieve a Noticeable Result."

You can also practice OFFICE YOGA without any

18

goal standard—without setting time limits, developing plans, or anticipating obstacles. Here's how this would work. Set goals, if you choose to, but don't be set on outcomes. Meanwhile, pay attention. In other words, during each exercise, watch, look, listen, and breathe deeply. When you are dealing with specific problems, you may even be able to heal yourself through spontaneous insights. This often works for me.

In any case, with practice, OFFICE YOGA will exercise all your body parts independently and synergistically —from head to toe, from angst to aura, and from sight to synchronicity.

I urge you to schedule OFFICE YOGA into your daily grind— and facilitate for yourself a shift from grind to grand.

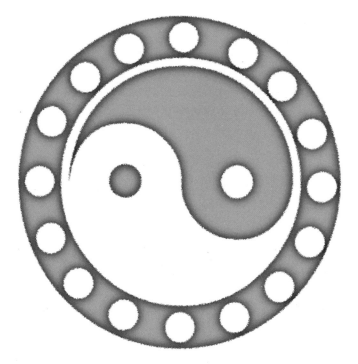

20

Yoga Eyes

Reading words that are at a fixed distance to the eye balls, such as when sitting for long periods at a computer screen, can reduce the elasticity of the eye muscles over the long-term. As with other parts of the body—whether it is the gluteus group mashed by the couch potato or the biceps of someone who never lifts a finger—unused muscles can atrophy

Computer workers can strengthen their eye muscles by focusing and re-focusing on objects that are at a variety of distances. For example, look up from your work and gaze out a window into the far distance, then shift your focus to something at close range, even a streak on the window glass itself. To strengthen the eye muscles easily and quickly, occasionally take a moment or two to visually toggle back and forth between a distant object and one close by. If you do this far focus/ close focus exercise on a regular basis—even for only 5 seconds—it will help to offset eye strain and the ultimate the deterioration of your vision.

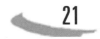

Another exercise that helps to strengthen the eyes is to occasionally soften or "fuzzy focus"—i.e. relax the muscles around your eyes and let your focus go "fuzzy." To assist you with this process, you will be reminded time and again in the OFFICE YOGA exercises to soften your gaze. Additionally, see the softened edges in the meditative illustrations on the left-hand pages in this book as examples of "fuzzy focus."

When we are stressed, our eye muscles automatically tense up. By softening the eyes, there is a corresponding relaxation in other parts of the body. For example, when my eye muscles relax, I feel a "letting go" of tension in my gut. It happens naturally. I also notice perceptual shifts. Soft eyes present a wide-angle view—bringing my perceptual world in closer and surrounding me with more choices and more intimacy.

Soft eyes also reflect receptive hearts—hearts that welcome intimacy. Tense eyes, on the other hand, perceive the world through a sharper, more telephoto-like lens, and this can distance us from others. Additionally, tight eyes reflect personalities that are out of touch with their own inner, gut feelings.

Yoga teaches us to see the world in new ways—and soft eyes help us to open up to new ideas like a wide-eyed child seeing the world for the very first time.

Puppet Strings

What does OFFICE YOGA have in common with Pinocchio? (Hint: It is not lying!) The answer is "puppet strings"—a metaphor used extensively in OFFICE YOGA to help you achieve the proper alignment and thus the greatest benefit from the exercises. For example, you will read an alignment direction such as, "Imagine that you can feel a puppet string attached to the crown of your head." Easy to picture and easy to achieve an excellent posture alignment. It is through these types of subtle self-corrections that the postures become most effective—and more pleasurable.

Be assured, however, that the puppet strings metaphor has nothing whatsoever to do with acting like a puppet with your boss—especially when it comes to getting permission to practice OFFICE YOGA!

If your boss or a co-worker comments when he or she sees you doing OFFICE YOGA, you can explain that these little stretches actually strengthen your body, clear your mind, and even increase your productivity.

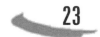

Yes! These exercises should, in fact, make your boss happy. But, just in case your boss or a co-worker doesn't see the light, you'll find excuses scattered throughout the text—such as, "I am contemplating the bottom line."

Alternately, if you feel like it, you may want to enlighten your co-workers about yoga. It is indeed a pragmatic science with 5,000 years of recorded history.

OFFICE YOGA is actually a self-care benefit package with user-friendly postures that make it possible to think more clearly, function more effectively, and remain free of pain while sitting and working for long hours at a desk or computer.

Breath and the Bliss Mist

Breath is the bottom line. Every breath we take is literally the moment we choose life. The Obituaries offer us this poignant reminder: "And then it was as if he just forgot to breathe..."*

Breath can help us to let go of tension and inflexibility. For this, exhale while you are stretching in the OFFICE YOGA exercises. Then, during inhalations hold your body more still.

The breath should be soft and gentle—always natural without tension or strain to it. Remember to breathe though your nose. This helps to prepare the air for your lungs, adjusting the temperature more closely to your body temperature and removing dust particles.

Breathing through the nose also slows down the breath—making it easier to observe your breath, your actions, and even your thoughts.

*Kennedy, Ed, "Watching death's door," 1/1/99, *Honolulu Advertiser.*

Use your full lung capacity—deeply inhaling, then exhaling every last ounce of stale air while you stretch further.

Breath can bring you great joy—Bliss. Slowly inhaling, deeply exhaling, activate your "observer," as if you are watching yourself from outside yourself rather than looking out through your own eyes. See if you can do both simultaneously—watching from outside and looking out from your eyes. Then see if you notice any changes in your perceptions.

As I explained on page 22, when my body gets enough oxygen and I am relaxed, my visual perception automatically shifts from a telephoto lens to a wide-angle view. Taking this one step further, the next thing that I observe is that my world looks misty, as if there is a soft-focus lens over my eyes. I think of this as the "Bliss Mist" because when mine arrives, I feel happy—for no reason! The Bliss Mist makes yoga (and everything else) easier, more effective—and fun, actually.

To arrive at the Bliss Mist, with these exercises follow the directions of each OFFICE YOGA exercise to the point where you start feeling like you want quit. The desire to quit is a clue that you are at the brink of the Bliss Mist. It can be caused by fatigue, or boredom, or maybe you just want to stop and you don't necessarily know or care why.

Don't quit. Don't give up immediately. Hang in there for another 5 seconds—inhaling fully while deepening your stretch with a long, slow exhalation. That's enough time to experience the Bliss Mist. It's short, but you can extend it.

Oxygen is one of the reasons for this. Stingy oxygenation can reduce our quality of life at every level: physical strength; concentration; memory; and emotional balance.

When we oxygenate our cells more fully, there are a number of perceptual shifts which can take place. Colors can become more vivid, thinking crisper, even hearts opening wider.

Breath can be a potent power to facilitate change. For this, set a goal during the brief pause after an exhalation and before an inhalation.

You can ride the momentum of your breath like a roller coaster ride to the depths of your being. You can do this while you practice OFFICE YOGA.

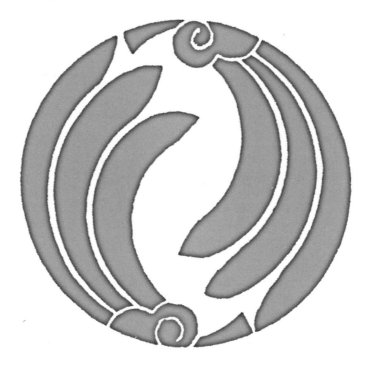

Perineum and Umbilical

OFFICE YOGA can be performed properly only when you activate your perineum and umbilical. The perineum-umbilical lock protects the body from injury while making the exercises easier to do.

The perineum can be found—on both men and women—between the bottom of the pubic bone and the bottom of the tail bone. The perineum consists of ligaments, nerves and muscles. Strengthening the perineum is a pleasurable sensation, so it is easy to remember once you start making this a habit.

> To identify your perineum, *stop the flow when you urinate.* To strengthen the perineum, practice squeezing and releasing (squeeze, 2, 3, release, 2, 3, squeeze, 2, 3, release, 2, 3) the muscles between the bottom of the pubic bone and the beginning of the tail bone.

The second part of the perineum-umbilical lock involves the muscles in the abdomen around the belly button, i.e., the umbilical.

> To activate the umbilical, pull in the belly button and say *haaa*.

The perineum and umbilical actions just described, when joined together, can take yoga to an exciting dimension of depth and intensity. Some of the benefits of the perineum-umbilical lock are:

- The sacrum adjusts itself and protects the low back from injury.

- A state of extraordinary balance is achieved. For example, I find I can stand on one leg without any other effort.

- Lung capacity increases. Breaths are more even and deeper—bringing additional oxygen to all the cells of the body.

- Every OFFICE Yoga posture instantly becomes more pleasurable—making them easier to do.

The perineum-umbilical lock is marked on all the full-sized illustrations of the OFFICE YOGA exercises with the following symbol ⊙.

Time

Hold each exercise for at least five seconds. If you can stay longer—up to three minutes—the exercises become considerably more effective, affording ample time to diffuse stress and restructure work habits.

During this five-second-to-three-minute period, while you are breathing slowly and stretching with each exhalation, also please notice if there is a desire to bolt. (It may be disguised as a sudden feeling of fatigue or disinterest.) In yoga, handling your desire to bolt will reveal to you how you are handling your life, including the limits of your physical stamina and mental preconceptions.

Is your desire to bolt part of a lifetime habit of dropping things when they require too much effort? If so, you can use OFFICE YOGA to re-ignite your energy for whatever purpose you desire—more money, a more peaceful life, attracting more love. Stamina in yoga is transferrable to stamina in other areas.

Perhaps start, if you have an urge to bolt, by

questioning yourself. You may want to ask yourself, *What does this stretch feel like? Is my body balanced side to side, front to back?* Yoga teaches us to observe our thoughts and feelings before they turn into actions. When we become occupied with the process of "observing," it is easier to relax in the stretches for extended periods.

You can also ease up in the stretches instead of bolting. Easing up extends the experience, and it shows that you are in control. Although some of the stretches may push the edges of your physical envelope, they should never cause serious pain or harm. By easing up, you will know that you are safe because you can stop whenever you want. You will find that easing up can also give you a second wind.

You may even discover whether or not your desire to bolt is a symptom of an old habit of trying to "control"—rather than adjusting to the flow of life.

By handling the desire to bolt, your comfort zone will expand, your enthusiasm will spring back, answers will bubble up from inside, and you will experience subtle changes in your thoughts and feelings. Handling your desire to bolt can offer you self-knowledge that converts into great value in the business world. Perseverance itself is an attribute with permanent assets—more valuable than gold bullion.

32

Strategies to Prolong Your Time

1. Ask yourself questions.

   Am I holding my breath?

   Is my body balanced side to side?

   Am I following all the instructions and performing the postures to the letter?

2. Knowing that you are in control, you can observe your desire to bolt.

3. Try backing off and see if this helps you to gather steam.

4. Examine patterns in your life that are similar to the desire to bolt when in the postures.

5. Observe subtle changes in perceptions, thoughts, and feelings.

6. When exhaling, push yourself—very gently—deeper into the poses. Stretch into the Bliss Mist.

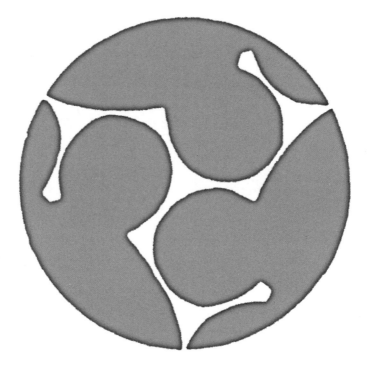

Symptom Chart

The following Symptom Chart may be useful for those who want to address specific problem areas. I have taken the liberty of collating all the symptoms into a single alphabetical list regardless of whether they are physical, mental, or emotional. My reasoning is that the body, mind, and emotions are intertwined in yoga —and the reality of this interrelatedness becomes more apparent as we practice yoga.

The symptoms on the left affect the back, brain, carpal tunnel, chest, circulation, coordination, digestion, dowager's hump, emotions, enthusiasm, eyes, face, feet, flexibility, gut feeling, headache, hips, immunity, legs, neck, shoulders, stress, thyroid and waistline. The suggested OFFICE YOGA exercises are alongside, and the exercises in **bold** are the most effective for that specific symptom or body part.

The lungs are not independently targeted because all the exercises increase the amount of fresh air intake. All the exercises work together synergistically— from the thighs to the eyes, from the nose to the toes.

Symptom/ Body Part	Exercise Bold = most effective	Page
Back	Alarm Neutralizer	87
	Cheerleader	95
	Frog Legs	129
	Homage	**77**
	Hump? What Hump?	**57**
	Rocky	69
	Telecom Twist	103
	Thumbs Down	73
Brain	Alarm Neutralizer	87
	Cheerleader	95
	Chin to Shin	**121**
	Face the Feet	133
	Frog Legs	129
	Homage	77
	Hump? What Hump?	57
	Monolith of Mastery	91
	Rocky	69
	Sky Stretch	125
	Swan Stretch	61
	Telecom Twist	103
	Thyroid Thrill	99
	Thumbs Down	73

Symptom/ Body Part	Exercise Bold = most effective	Page
Circulation	Alarm Neutralizer	87
	Cheerleader	95
	Chin to Shin	**121**
	Face the Feet	133
	Homage	77
	Hump? What Hump?	57
	Telecom Twist	103
	Toe Ups	**117**
Coordination	Alarm Neutralizer	87
	Bow and Arrow	65
	Cheerleader	**95**
	Hump? What Hump?	57
	Monolith of Mastery	91
	Rocky	69
	Toe Ups	**117**
Digestion	Alarm Neutralizer	87
	Chin to Shin	121
	Frog Legs	129
	Monolith of Mastery	**91**
	Sky Stretch	**125**
	Telecom Twist	103

Symptom/ Body Part	Exercise Bold = most effective	Page
Eyes	**Bow and Arrow**	**65**
	Cheerleader	95
	Focus Time	**107**
	Poker Face	111
	Rocky	69
	Telecom Twist	103
	Thumbs Down	73
Face	Face the Feet	133
	Hump? What Hump?	57
	Poker Face	**111**
	Swan Stretch	61
Feet	Homage	77
	Toe Ups	**117**
Flexibility	Alarm Neutralizer	87
	Chin to Shin	121
	Face the Feet	133
	Frog Legs	**129**
	Homage	77
	Telecom Twist	**103**
	Toe Ups	117

Symptom/ Body Part	Exercise Bold = most effective	Page
Gut Feeling	Chin to Shin	121
	Face the Feet	133
	Monolith of Mastery	91
	Sky Stretch	**125**
	Telecom Twist	**103**
Headache	Bow and Arrow	65
	Homage	77
	Thumbs Down	73
	Rocky	69
	Swan Stretch	**61**
Hips	Alarm Neutralizer	87
	Chin to Shin	121
	Face the Feet	133
	Frog Legs	129
	Homage	**77**
Immunity	Alarm Neutralizer	87
	Cheerleader	95
	Face the Feet	133
	Homage	**77**
	Thyroid Thrill	99

Symptom/ Body Part	Exercise Bold = most effective	Page
Legs	Chin to Shin	121
	Face the Feet	133
	Frog Legs	129
	Toe Ups	**117**
Neck	Bow and Arrow	65
	Homage	77
	Hump? What Hump?	57
	Swan Stretch	**61**
	Thumbs Down	**73**
	Thyroid Thrill	99
Shoulders	Alarm Neutralizer	87
	Bow and Arrow	65
	Cheerleader	95
	Homage	**77**
	Hump? What Hump?	**57**
	Monolith of Mastery	91
	Palm Press Project	81
	Rocky	69
	Sky Stretch	125
	Thumbs Down	**73**
	Thyroid Thrill	99

Symptom/ Body Part	Exercise Bold = most effective	Page
Stress	**Alarm Neutralizer**	**87**
	Bow and Arrow	65
	Cheerleader	95
	Homage	77
	Monolith of Mastery	91
	Palm Press Project	81
	Rocky	69
	Sky Stretch	125
	Swan Stretch	61
	Telecom Twist	**103**
Thyroid	Bow and Arrow	65
	Cheerleader	95
	Swan Stretch	61
	Thyroid Thrill	99
Waistline	Alarm Neutralizer	87
	Homage	**77**
	Monolith of Mastery	**91**
	Sky Stretch	125
	Telecom Twist	**103**
Wrists	(See: Carpal Tunnel Stress)	

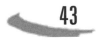

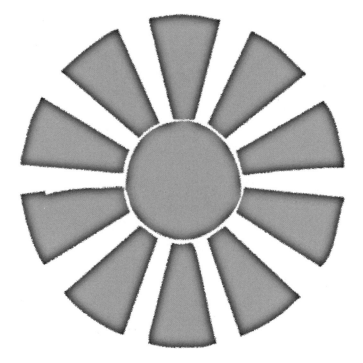

Modify, Modify, Modify

Are you a right-handed person using a right-hand keyboard and mouse? If so, does your body—as mine once did—slouch towards the right?

Slouching must be corrected—for us to attain optimum health and clear thinking—which is what the Office Yoga exercises are geared to do. Slouching torques the neck, and this impairs blood flow to the brain and slows down the thinking process. Not attractive. Not lucrative. Not interesting.

It is yoga which has given me awareness of imbalances in my body from side to side. Optimum productivity comes automatically as both sides of the body gain in strength and flexibility—and the whole is greater than the sum of all the parts.

My right thumb gave up during the final edit of Jet Smarter. I had been in the habit of hitting the spacebar with my right thumb and at that point, every thumb tap caused pain.

I had to complete JET SMARTER at maximum speed (luckily there were back orders), so I immediately began to train myself to tap the spacebar with my left thumb. Talk about feeling clumsy! But pain (and back orders) can be a great motivator to try new things. I kept telling myself, *You trained the right thumb way back when, and now you can certainly train your left thumb.* During this time, my right thumb kept trying to race for the spacebar first, and eventually, my right index finger took over the task, without my conscious command. *Air traffic control, wake up!*

At the same time, I was trying to train my left thumb. I moved the mouse over to the left side of my keyboard. I am now clicking a right-handed mouse with my left middle finger or sometimes the index finger. I like to change over to strengthen both fingers.

This is an example of "Modify, Modify, Modify." OFFICE YOGA exercises are designed to be modified. As you do each exercise, you will know—by what you cannot do—how you need to modify the exercise. Keep in mind that while it is important to feel your muscles stretch, there definitely should be no intense pain anywhere and especially not in the knees or low back. If you have not stretched in a long while, or you find an exercise too difficult, consider it too advanced for awhile and wait until you've made some progress before attempting it again.

46

As you modify each exercise, your practice will become unique and you will find that your range of motion—less or greater than those portrayed in the illustrations—is always changing as it is affected by your "edges" built up by a lifetime of actions, emotions, decisions, experiences, and injuries.

A word about injuries—today there are trendy aerobic yoga styles pushing students to power past old injuries. I believe this can be harmful. In the past, this type of practice has caused me harm. I do not advise people to power past old injuries, and, once I made this decision in my own practice, I got a lot more back from my yoga without long periods of downtime.

Body parts that have been previously injured and repaired may need special care—perhaps even for a lifetime. On a positive note, we can learn from previous injuries how to listen to subtle bodily signals and how to modify our behavior accordingly.

If you don't already do this, here's how you can start listening to your body: When sitting at your desk, occasionally do a mental scan to become aware of where you are tense (jaw, neck, shoulders, etc.). Then release this tension. You may need to mentally send a message to "let go" and release a knot of tension or resistance quite a number of times when you first become aware of it. But persistence will bring results.

 47

Next, check occasionally to see that both sides of your body carry your weight equally—either on your feet (if you are standing) or on your butt and feet (if you are in your chair).

Finally, please do not assume that any limits you are experiencing are permanent.

For yoga novices, OFFICE YOGA will start you on the yoga track, so that if you decide you want to probe deeper, you can join a yoga class armed with the confidence that comes from already understanding the basics of yoga.

Be aware, however, that most classes don't spend enough time holding/breathing in each exercise—a vital esoteric premise of yoga (p.31, Time). Yoga, without holding still long enough to dive into the knot of resistance and face it as the bully it is, is like eating bread which hasn't had time to rise.

But classes are a great way to learn a variety of exercises (postures), and this will offer you the opportunity to find out which ones you like best. Then, you can do them on your own for long periods, i.e., 5 seconds to 3 minutes. This is long enough to have an internal experience. (p.25, Breath and the Bliss Mist).

Classes also offer the valuable opportunity to get feedback on your alignment from an instructor.

However, I most emphatically recommend that no matter what is being taught or suggested, you should feel free to modify it in any way you want. We all need to modify our behavior according to our past injuries, innate flexibility, and our own internal guidance.

Once you learn to modify the exercises, you will find that Office Yoga is adaptable to other environments. For example, you can easily do the exercises in an airport transit lounge prior to boarding your flight. This will help you get over jetlag. (In-flight exercises for jetlag and healthy flying are available in my book Jet Smarter: The Air Traveler's Rx.)

Once you begin to practice and get in the habit of modifying, you will think of more ways to adapt these stretches in other situations in your daily life. As you push the edges of your physical flexibility, you will find a greater emotional balance comes to you naturally, as well. As emotional edges broaden, they automatically become less sharp—and they are less likely to hurt you and others.

Certainly one of the most wonderful and magical benefits of yoga is that we become more aware of our responses—the entire palette of responses available to us—before reacting to and coloring our world.

49

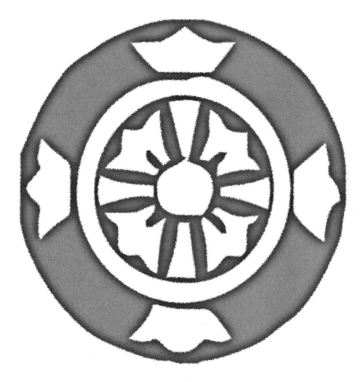

The Place

It is best to do OFFICE YOGA in a well-ventilated place with as much fresh air as possible. Toxic chemical vapors near where you work can damage your lungs, as well as the nervous, reproductive, and immune systems—and contribute to stress, pain, and lack of productivity and efficiency. Then, there's the additional task of eliminating these toxins from the body. (From my book, NONI: Aspirin of the Ancients: "Poisons can be removed. I drink a lot of water, take hot saunas and baths, and eat certain herbs such as noni to help eliminate poisons from my body.")

So, put the fax machine and copy machine on the other side of the room, or better yet, in a separate room from where you sit most of the time, whenever this is possible.

A further caution about your work place is body-considerate (ergonomic) furniture. Be willing to make adjustments to the location of your desk as well as with the height of your keyboard, monitor, and chair.

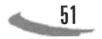

On the facing page you'll find a list of ergonomic criteria for consideration to help your body function optimally while doing computer work. Ultimately, however, no one can tell you every detail about how to set up your work-space—*you* need to tune-in for yourself.

In addition to your computer set up, wear clothes that are truly comfortable. They should be breathable, and suitable for sitting for long hours especially after eating when the center of the body tends to swell up. I love wearing organic cotton clothing; I can feel the difference in my nervous system compared to wearing other fabrics and also those with sizing. (Sizing is made from formaldehyde, which is a neurotoxin.)

Next, for the few moments you practice OFFICE YOGA, mentally move aside all thoughts about your work. Even if it's just for a minute or two, you will find that creating an internal, quiet space will provide you with a valuable respite—from which you will be able to return to your office tasks with renewed energy and, often, with an increased flow of creativity.

You can also create private auditory space by allowing the sounds around you to become part of your practice—even the hum of the fluorescents, or the tap of a keyboard nearby—people talking, phones ringing. I like to imagine that all this background cacophony is a techie-new-world symphony tuning up.

Ergonomic Work Station Criteria

- The monitor has minimal glare so that you can look at the monitor without squinting. The height and angle of the monitor allow you to see the screen without hunching over, looking up, or torquing your neck to one side.

- The keyboard allows your hands, wrists, arms, and shoulders to work without tension. You may need to change the keyboard distance and height—below elbow height is more comfortable for the wrists and shoulders. Resting my wrists on a wrist rest helps a lot.

- Your feet can rest firmly on the floor without stressing your legs. Can you take off your shoes while you sit at the computer? Wiggle your toes from time to time to stimulate the blood flow.

- The chair enables you to sit comfortably with good posture.

- Your clothes are loose and do not dig into your flesh or leave marks on your skin.

Reduce Pain

Pain can be a powerful teacher. Pain teaches us to appreciate moments that are free of pain. It determines our character once we realize nobody will put up with a complainer. Pain reminds us that we are mortal—and this changes everything.

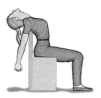

Hump? What Hump?
Neck Pain / Deformed Spine......57

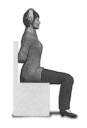

Swan Stretch
Headache / Neck Pain...............61

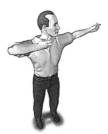

Bow and Arrow
Headache / Poor Circulation...65

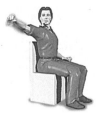

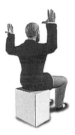

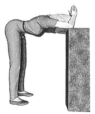

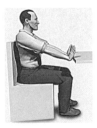

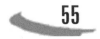

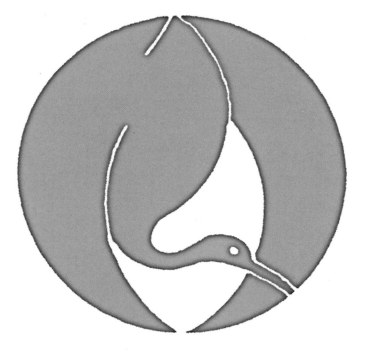

Hump? What Hump?

A 30-second yoga moment

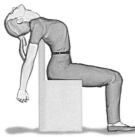

Consider This

Sitting hunched over a computer can create a deformity at the base of the neck—the so-called "dowager's hump."

Rationale

"Hump? What Hump?" will reduce and can even eliminate the dowager's hump.

Time to Achieve a Noticeable Result

Two months, when done once/day for 30 seconds.

Added Perk

Alleviates a double chin.

How To Do "Hump? What Hump?"

- It's best to do "Hump? What Hump?" in a chair with a solid back (not a tilting back). So, sit with your feet hip-width apart. Position the heels of your feet directly under the backs of your knees.

- Balance your upper body with equal weight on both sides of your butt. Hang your arms over the back of the chair. Interlace your fingers and join your palms together. ⊙Activate your perineum-umbilical lock.

- Keeping your breastbone lifted, breathe naturally and drop your head back. Look at the ceiling with a softened focus and notice your peripheral vision.

- Lower your shoulders. Stretch your hands away from your body. Slowly open and close your mouth and stick out your tongue.

- Close your mouth and carefully return to an upright position. The next time you do " Hump? What Hump?" change the interlace on your fingers so the other thumb is on top. This will help to balance the right and left hemispheres of the brain while strengthening both sides of the body.

In Brief

- ◈ Join hands behind back.
- ◈ Pull hands away and up.
- ◈ Lift chest.
- ◈ Lengthen spine.
- ◈ Breathe deeply.

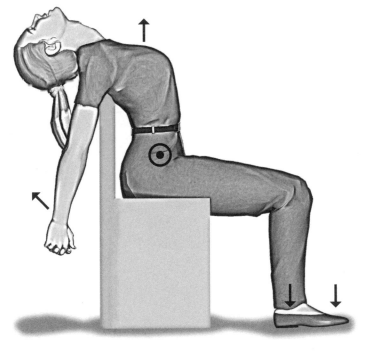

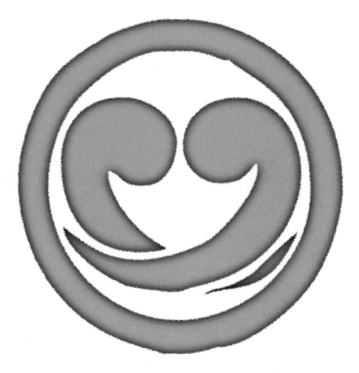

Swan Stretch

A 1-minute yoga moment

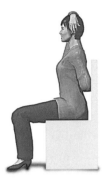

Consider This

When the neck is torqued in one direction for extended periods, for example, while typing and referring to notes, this can reduce both cerebrospinal fluid and oxygen to the brain—and result in tension headaches

Rationale

"Swan Stretch" helps to un-torque the neck.

Time to Achieve a Noticeable Result

One week, when done twice/day for 1 minute.

Added Perks

Smooths the skin of the neck.

How To Do "Swan Stretch"

- Balance your upper body with equal weight on both sides of your butt. ⊙Activate your perineum-umbilical lock.

- Exhaling, bend your left arm and place it behind your waist with your palm touching the back of your chair. Your left elbow is close to your waist.

- With your right hand, reach over the top of your head and cover your left ear. Then, gently tug your head and tilt your right ear towards your right shoulder. Extend your lower lip in an exaggerated pout.

- Inhale deeply and exhale fully, then return your mouth to a smile and your head to its normal vertical alignment. As you bring your left arm back to your side, take a moment to picture a swan taking off. Swans are admired for their graceful necks—as this exercise will help to restore grace to your neck.

- Repeat "Swan Stretch" with your right hand behind your back and your left hand on your right ear tilting your left ear towards your left shoulder. This will help to balance the right and left hemispheres of the brain while strengthening both sides of your neck.

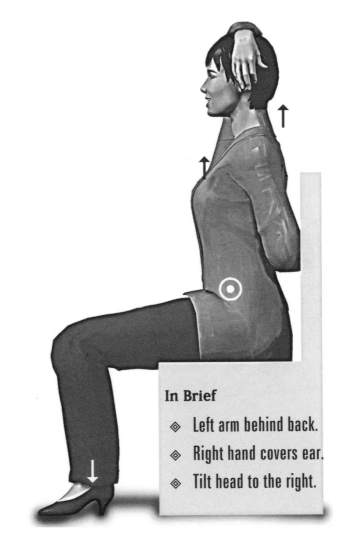

In Brief

◈ Left arm behind back.

◈ Right hand covers ear.

◈ Tilt head to the right.

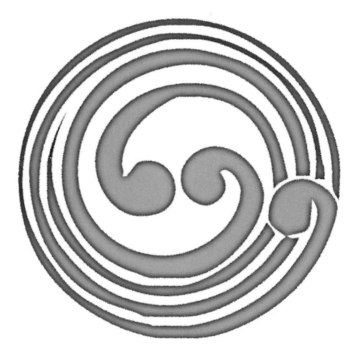

Bow and Arrow

A 20-second yoga moment

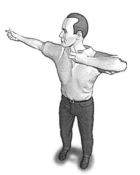

Consider This

Sitting for long hours—using only the hands and the mind and not moving the rest of the body—can lead to impaired bodily circulation and coordination.

Rationale

Taoist monks purportedly practiced "Bow and Arrow" to exercise the body while spending long hours in quiet meditation.

Time to Achieve a Noticeable Result

Eight weeks, when done once/day for 20 seconds.

Added Perk

Improves vision (externally and internally).

How To Do "Bow and Arrow"

- "Bow and Arrow" can be perfected seated or standing. Either way, be sure your upper-body weight is evenly supported on both sides.

- Lift your neck as if you feel a puppet string attached to the crown of your head. Raise your elbows to shoulder height with a puppet string attacked to each elbow. ⊙Activate your perineum-umbilical lock.

- Your right arm becomes the arrow; as you straighten your right arm, point your right index finger (the arrow tip). Lift your right thumb; imagine your right thumbnail is a computer monitor and on this screen you now see, in perfect detail and clarity, a goal that you wish to attain.

- Your left hand pulls back the bowstring. Breathe deeply and, on any exhalation, release the arrow.

- See the arrow fly. See the arrow reach your goal.

- Next time, do "Bow & Arrow," with the left hand as the arrow and the right hand pulling the bowstring. This will help to balance the right and left hemispheres of the brain and improve vision in both eyes.

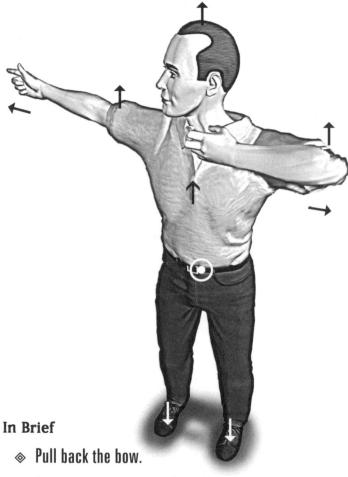

In Brief

- ◈ Pull back the bow.
- ◈ See a target or a mental goal.
- ◈ Release the arrow.

67

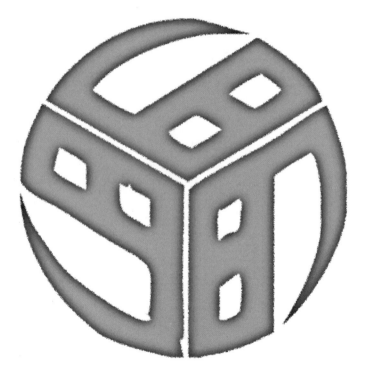

Rocky

A 10-second yoga moment

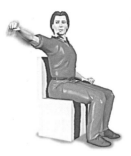

Consider This

Concentrating at a computer, the upper body may slump forwards and this can cause back strain and shoulder pain.

Rationale

"Rocky" strengthens the upper back and shoulders.

Time to Achieve a Noticeable Result

One week, when done twice/day for 10 seconds.

Added Perk

Alleviates drooping eyelids.

How To Do "Rocky"

- If the arms on your chair impede your elbows in this exercise, you can *scooch* forwards or stand. Sitting or standing, your feet are hip-width apart.

- Your hands are relaxed in your lap (or, standing, at your sides) in loose fists with fingers up (or forwards). ⊙ Activate your perineum-umbilical. Lift your neck as if a puppet string were attached to the crown of your head. Breathing deeply, feel your lungs expand equally on both sides of your chest.

- Raise your eyebrows. Watching your right fist, punch to the right, turning your fist over so the knuckles are up. Relax your eyebrows and return your fist to your lap (or side), again with palm up.

- Raise your eyebrows again and, watching your left fist, punch to the left, turning your fist over so the knuckles are up. Then lower your eyebrows and return the left fist back to your lap (or side).

- Punch several more times. With each punch, raise your eyebrows and exhale. Find a punching rhythm. Build up energy. Be quick and precise like Rocky.

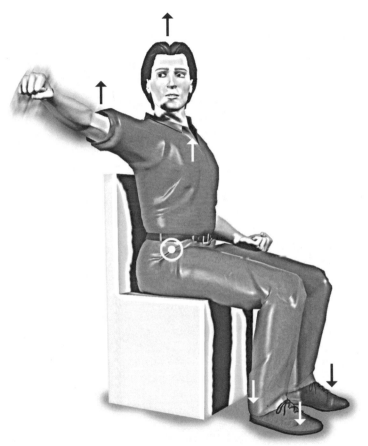

In Brief

◈ Punch and your fist turns over.

◈ Follow your fist with your eyes.

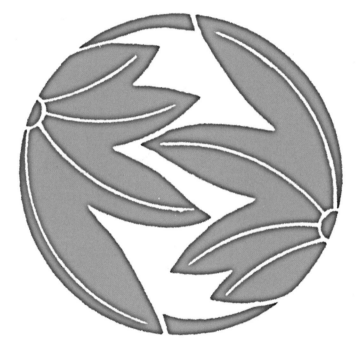

Thumbs Down

A 40-second yoga moment

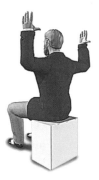

Consider This

Working for long hours at a desk may cause the upper body to slump forward, which could result in neck pain and foggy thinking.

Rationale

"Thumbs Down" helps the body to maintain good posture, relieving neck pain and foggy thinking.

Time to Achieve a Noticeable Result

One week, when done once/day for 40 seconds.

Added Perk

Tones the bags under the eyes.

How To Do "Thumbs Down"

- Sit with your feet hip-width apart. Balance equal weight on both sides of your butt. ⊙ Activate your perineum-umbilical. Your palms are on both sides of your head; your thumbs about the level of the ears. As you stretch your thumbs back and down, try to keep the distance between your elbows the same as the distance between your hands.

- Allow your elbows to rotate forward. Inhale deeply and exhale fully feeling your lungs expand on both sides and in front and back of your chest. Exhaling, lift your neck as if you feel a puppet string attached to the crown of your head press your thumbs down.

- Turn to look at one of your hands and, focus on the tiny lines in your palm. Turn your head 180 degrees and focus on the other palm. Then, close your eyes and imagine you can feel your brain waves rebounding between your palms.

- The next time you do "Thumbs Down" look at the other hand first. This will help to balance the right and left hemispheres of the brain while toning the bags under the eyes.

74

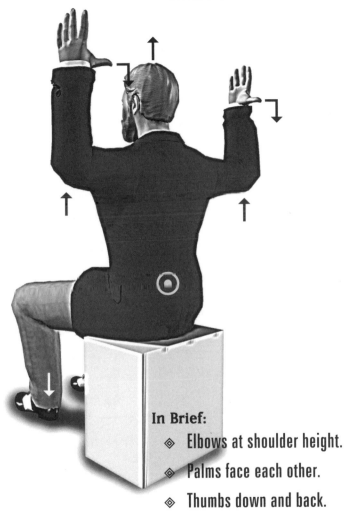

In Brief:

◈ Elbows at shoulder height.

◈ Palms face each other.

◈ Thumbs down and back.

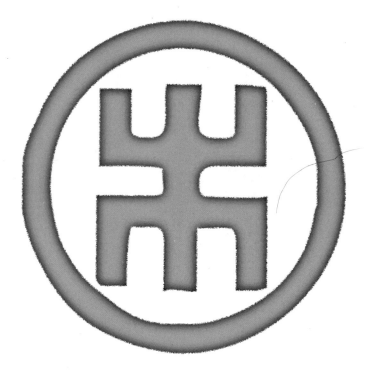

Homage

A 1-minute yoga moment

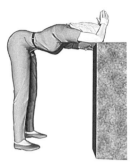

Consider This

Sitting for long hours at a desk may cause neck, upper back and shoulder pains.

Rationale

"Homage" stretches and relieves tightness in the neck, upper back and shoulders. This is my favorite OFFICE YOGA exercise.

Time to Achieve a Noticeable Result

Two weeks, when done twice/day for 1 minute.

Added Perk

Narrows the waistline.

How To Do "Homage"

- Stand up. Your toes face forward. Place your elbows on your desk or console and back up until your feet are below your hipbones. Wiggle each toe independently, then press your toes and heels down, and broaden your footprints.

- ⊙ Activate your perineum-umbilical. Relax your forehead on the desk or console between your biceps; your palms touching.

- Your back is flat. The top of your head stretches forward and your hips stretch back, while at the same time broaden the space between your shoulder blades and lengthen your sides

- Lift your kneecaps by tightening your thigh muscles. Try to equalize your weight on all five points (two feet, two elbows, and forehead).

- Inhale deeply and exhale fully feeling your lungs expand equally on both sides and in front and back of your chest.

- With each inhalation as your lungs expand, expand your expectations, your hopes, and your dreams.

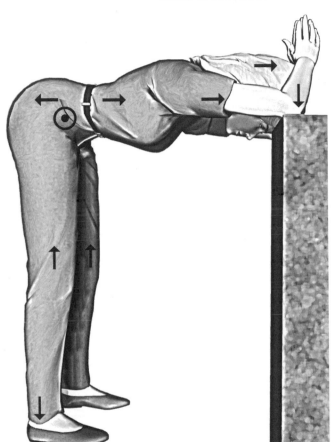

In Brief

◈ Feet hip-width apart.

◈ Lengthen torso.

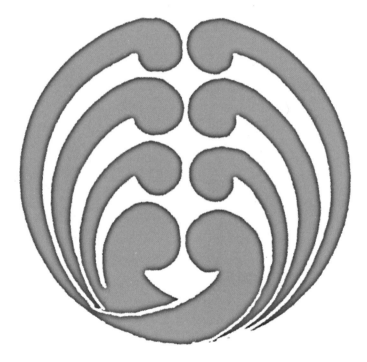

Palm Press Project

A 30-second yoga moment

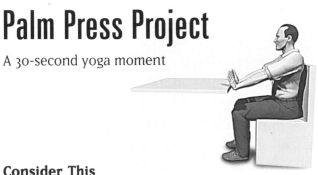

Consider This

Typing can injure the ligaments on the underside of the wrists, and this affects the arms, shoulders and back. If your wrists are swollen or painful, it is also important to practice "Alarm Neutralizer," "Bow and Arrow," "Hump? What Hump?," "Monolith of Mastery," "Rocky," "Sky Stretch" and "Thumbs Down."

Rationale

"Palm Press Project" helps to heal carpal tunnel stress.

Time to Achieve at Noticeable Result

Two weeks, when done four times/day for 30 seconds.

Added Perk

Firms the chest muscles.

How To Do "Palm Press Project"

- Your feet are hip-width apart. Your upper body is balanced with equal weight on both sides of your butt. ☉ Activate your perineum-umbilical lock. Lift your neck and breastbone. Inhale deeply and exhale fully, feeling your lungs expand equally on both sides and in front and back of your chest.

- Place your hands shoulder-width apart and perpendicular to the edge of your desk. Your elbows are straight; so if you are too close to the edge of your desk move your chair back or practice "Palm Press Project" standing up.

- The insides of your elbows face each other. Straighten your fingers and press the base of your fingers with equal pressure from pinky to thumb, bending your elbows slightly as necessary and feeling your pectoral muscles contract. Carefully modify hand placements and pressure rhythms. Have fun!

- If your wrists are painful, take time to identify other activities throughout your day that may be stressing them. Support your wrists at the computer and keep corporate tunnel syndrome at arm's length.

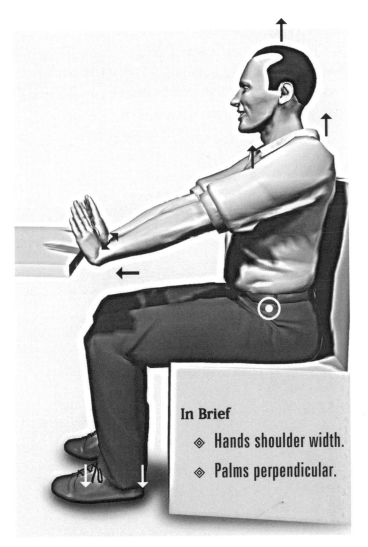

In Brief

◈ Hands shoulder width.

◈ Palms perpendicular.

Improve Efficiency

You have a constant flow of ideas. You work faster, cleaner, make a better product, all the while having fun. You are not a well-oiled machine, but a person who takes pride in what you do.

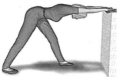

Alarm Neutralizer

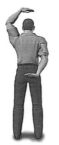

Monolith of Mastery

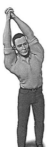

Cheerleader

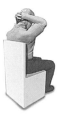

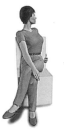

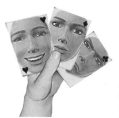

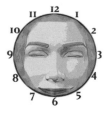

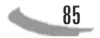

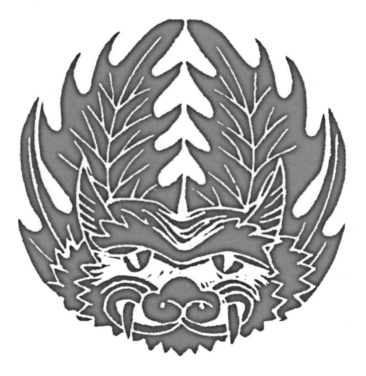

Alarm Neutralizer

A 45-second yoga moment

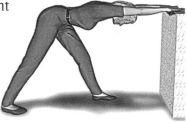

Consider This

When things aren't working out as we had hoped they would, we sometimes feel a sense of alarm. Excessive alarm can lead to exhaustion of the adrenals.

Rationale

"Alarm Neutralizer" stretches the mid-back where the adrenal glands reside (just above the waist at both sides). Stretching the mid-back brings oxygenated blood to help the adrenals function optimally, i.e., to maintain calmness in crises and, hopefully, eliminate the need to take drugs for anxiety.

Time to Achieve a Noticeable Result

Eight weeks, when done once/day for 45 seconds.

Added Perk

Narrows the waistline.

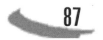
87

How To Do "Alarm Neutralizer"

- Stand up and place your palms on a flat surface such as a desk or shelf. Step backward and stretch your spine parallel to the floor.

- Your feet are one big step apart, both feet facing forward. Both hips face forward (adjust the front hip back and the back hip forward).

- Lift your kneecaps by flexing your thigh muscles. ⊙ Activate your perineum-umbilical.

- Stretch your fingertips forward. Press down the heels of your hands, then pull your body slightly back, stretching your wrists and underarms.

- Check that your weight is equally supported on both hands and both feet. Broaden the space between your shoulder blades and stretch from the top of your head to your tailbone. Soften your gaze.

- Switch your feet so the other foot is in back; the side with the foot in back gets the benefit of more fresh blood flow to the adrenal area.

Excuse to Boss

"I'm contemplating the bottom line."

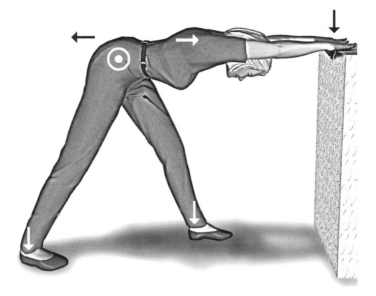

In Brief

⬦ Take several steps back.

⬦ Lengthen from crown to tail bone.

⬦ Broaden between the shoulder blades.

⬦ Soften your gaze.

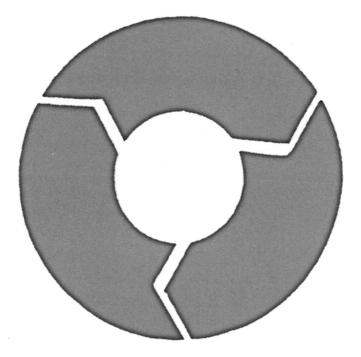

Monolith of Mastery

A 30-second yoga moment

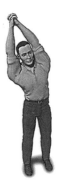

Consider This

Working long hours can be stressful, especially when there is tension in the workplace.

Rationale

If tension is your companion, do "Monolith of Mastery." Then, when you get pushed by forces and perspectives, you won't get knocked over.

Time to Achieve a Noticeable Result

Four weeks, when done once/day for 30 seconds.

Added Perk

A big stretch gives you an aura of confidence.

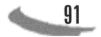

How To Do "Monolith of Mastery"

- Stand with your feet hip-width apart, balancing your weight equally on both feet.

- Lift your kneecaps by flexing your thigh muscles.

- Reach up and interlace your fingers. Stretch up with imaginary puppet strings attached to your fingers and breastbone. If possible, your palms are touching and your head is between your biceps.

- ⊙ Activate your perineum/umbilical and tilt your upper body towards the left. Press down with your right heel and elongate your right side from your heel to your fingers, breathing deeply. Soft gaze.

- Return to center, change the interlace on your fingers so the other thumb is on top.

- Stretch to the right. Press down with your left heel and elongate your left side, breathing deeply.

- Come back to center. If you have noticed that one side is weaker, do that side first next time and also more often, to try to bring your body into balance.

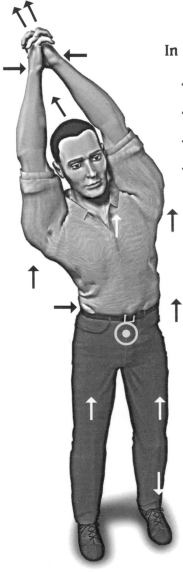

In Brief

- ◈ Head between biceps.
- ◈ Palms touching.
- ◈ Pull arms to one side.
- ◈ Gaze soft.

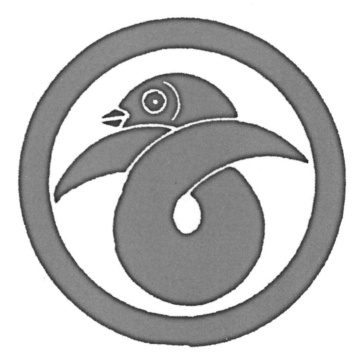

Cheerleader

A 20-second yoga moment

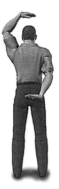

Consider This

When the body is relatively inert for hours at the computer (with only the hands, eyes and mind activated), all your senses can become dulled.

Rationale:

"Cheerleader" brings vibrancy to the senses; this speeds up your reaction times in tasking and in thinking.

Time to Achieve a Noticeable Result

Two weeks, when done once/day for 20 seconds.

Added Perk

Subtle integration between feelings and behavior.

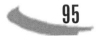

How To Do "Cheerleader"

- Stand with your toes facing forward and your knees slightly bent directly over your toes. Your weight is equally supported on both feet.

- With eyes closed or open, rub your hands until you feel heat in your palms.

- Mindful of this heat (this energy) passing between your palms, exhale slowly and pull your hands apart. Your left arm reaches up and the left hand (above your head) faces down. Inhale.

- Your right arm reaches down and the palm faces up (near your tailbone). Exhale. Relax your wrists and elbows. Breathe deeply and stretch your spine upwards, visualizing a puppet string attached to the crown of your head.

- Feel energy flowing between your palms, then circulating to your spine, into your torso, and to all your vital organs.

- Rub your hands together again; balance with one more "Cheerleader"; this time with the right hand on top.

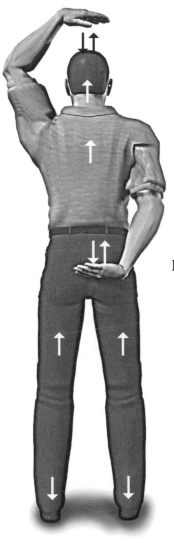

In Brief

◈ Top palm faces down.

◈ Bottom palm faces up.

◈ Feel the energy flow.

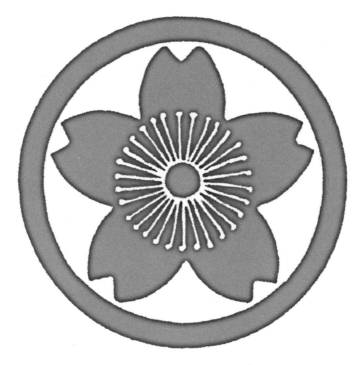

Thyroid Thrill

A 20-second yoga moment

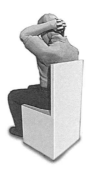

Consider This

If your work environment requires you to muzzle your voice, "Thyroid Thrill" will help to release pent-up and potentially toxic thought-forms (mental images).

Rationale

"Thyroid Thrill" helps to balance the emotions with natural hormonal secretions of the thyroid gland.

Time to Achieve a Noticeable Result

Two months, when done once/day for 20 seconds.

Added Perk

Stimulates the libido.

How To Do "Thyroid Thrill"

- Balance your upper body with equal weight on both sides of your butt. Your feet are flat on the ground; position the heels directly under the backs of your knees. Your back is straight; align your shoulders above your hipbones.

- Interlace your fingers behind your head at the base of your skull. ☉ Activate your perineum-umbilical lock, and relax your jaw and tongue.

- Squeeze your elbows together. Focus with your mind's eye on your thyroid gland (two lobes on either side of the windpipe below the Adam's apple).

- Breathe deeply and with each exhalation stretch your neck up, imaging a puppet string attached to the top of your head.

- Create a little resistance between your hands (pushing forward) and your head (pushing back and up).

- Feel the thyroid thrill as it secretes its hormonal juice. Tune into emotional shifts prompted by the thyroid's juiciness.

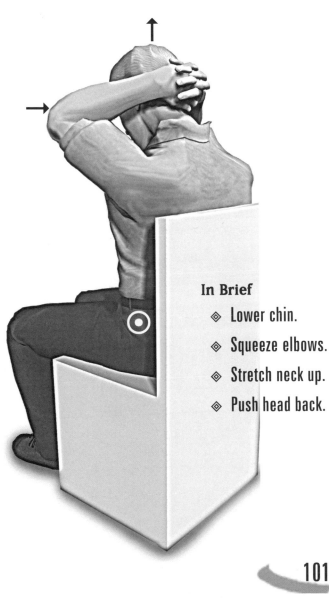

In Brief

◈ Lower chin.

◈ Squeeze elbows.

◈ Stretch neck up.

◈ Push head back.

101

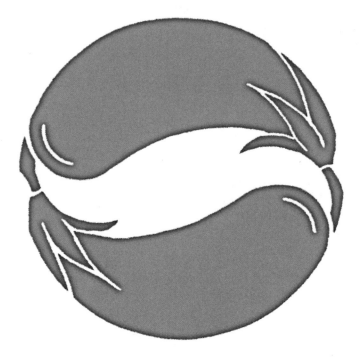

Telecom Twist

A 30-second yoga moment

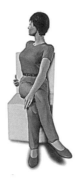

Consider This

When the body is virtually locked in one position all day hunched over a desk or computer, pain can ensue in the back and shoulders.

Rationale

"Telecom Twist" increases your range of motion and depth of perception. Our world of resources is everywhere around us; with a flexible spine, opportunities are easier to see and embrace.

Time to Achieve a Noticeable Result

One week, when done twice/day for 30 seconds.

Added Perk

a) Physical: flattens the abdomen. b) Subtle: strengthens your "center" and gut feelings.

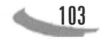

How To Do "Telecom Twist"

- Balance your upper body with equal weight on both sides of your butt. Your feet are flat on the ground; position the heels directly under the backs of your knees. ⊙ Activate your perineum-umbilical lock.

- Your back is straight; align your shoulders above your hipbones. Your arms are relaxed at your sides.

- Cross your right leg over your left. Your left hand rests on your right knee or thigh. Your right hand reaches behind and grasps the back of your chair. Twist to the right, your body first and your head next.

- Breathe deeply and with each exhalation stretch your neck up, imaging a puppet string attached to the crown of your head. Close your eyes and take a few breaths, deepening the twist and lifting your neck with each exhalation.

- Untwist, come back to center, then cross your left leg over your right. Your left hand reaches behind as you twist to the left, your body first and your head next.

- Come back to center. Back to work.

104

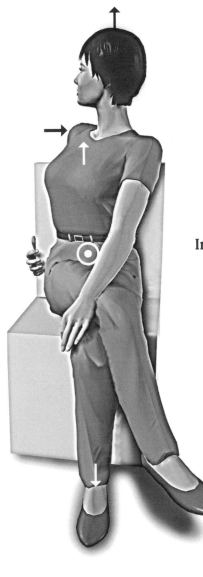

In Brief

- ◈ Right leg over left.
- ◈ Left elbow straight.
- ◈ Twist tall.

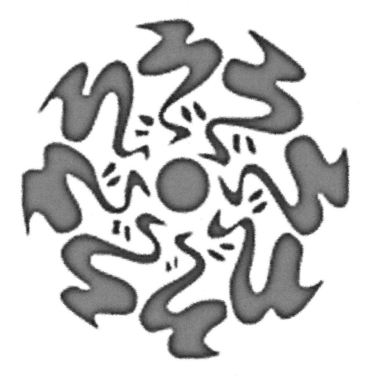

Focus Time

A 1-minute yoga moment

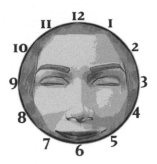

Consider This

Eye muscles tend to lose elasticity when you continually focus them at a fixed distance, such as when reading printed matter or the computer screen.

Rationale

"Focus Time" helps to revive the eye muscles.

Time to Achieve a Noticeable Result

Two weeks, when done three times/day for 1 minute.

Added Perk

See the motives behind people's actions.

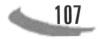

How To Do "Focus Time"

- Balance your upper body with equal weight on both sides of your butt. Your feet are flat on the ground; position the heels directly under the backs of your knees. Your back is straight; align your shoulders above your hipbones. Feel puppet strings tugging the crown of your head and your breastbone.

- **Eye Exercise 1.** With eyes open or closed, imagine a clock around the perimeter of your eye sockets. Focus on any number on this imaginary clock, then let your eyes alight around the clock face from one number to the next. Cut corners, if you like, but be sure to touch down on all the numbers. Inhale or exhale as you bring each new number into focus. Exhale fully each time.

- **Eye Exercise 2.** Toggle your focus between a near object, such as your finger held up in front of you, and another object further away, such as the horizon when looking out a window.

- **Eye Therapy.** Reduce eyestrain by softening your ambient interior light to a comfortable intensity and by wearing sunglasses in bright daylight.

108

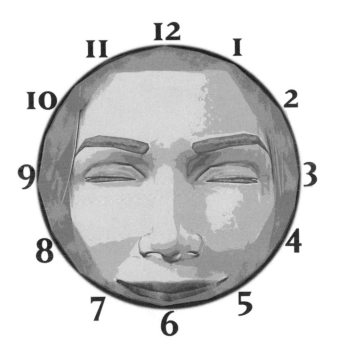

In Brief

◈ Imagine a clock around your eyes.

◈ Shift your forcus from number to number.

◈ Breathe deelply as you change numbers.

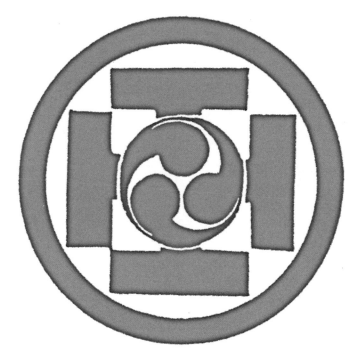

Poker Face

A 10-second yoga moment

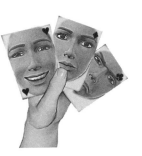

Consider This

Glancing at your mirror, do you see an expression you would like to encounter every day at work?

Rationale

"Poker Face" helps you to master your facial expression and be instantly more attractive.

Time to Achieve a Noticeable Result

Two weeks, when done six times/day for 10 seconds.

Added Perk

Opens doors—socially and professionally.

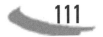

How To Do "Poker Face"

- Your feet are balanced evenly on the floor. Lift your neck as if you feel a puppet string attached to the crown of your head.

- ⊙ Inhale deeply activating the perineum-umbilical lock and feeling your lungs expand equally on both sides and in front and back of your chest.

- Exhale fully as you slacken all the muscles on your face—mouth, eyes, brow, and jaw. Breathe deeply at your own comfortable pace. Your tongue is flipped up and back so that the bottom of the tongue touches the top of your pallet and the tip of the tongue is relaxed near your throat.

- Do a mental scan of your body to see how different the perineum-umbilical lock feels when all the muscles in the face are soft and relaxed.

- Think about what it means to "save face." Enter the soft center of yourself exhaling deeply and completely, inhaling slowly. Breathe placidly amid the noise and haste. Once you have sovereignty over your own face, you gain a big advantage in any negotiation.

112

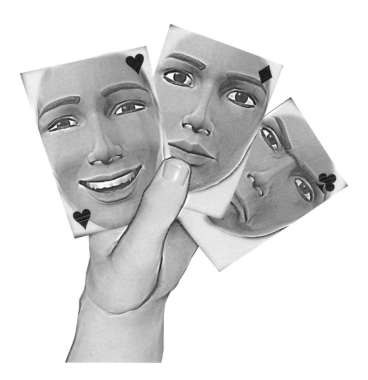

In Brief

◈ Relax your face.

◈ Breathe placidly amid the noise and haste.

Increase Productivity

The bottom line about productivity is love. Do you love what you do? Spending long hours at work is easy when you are enthralled. And love stimulates the immune system. When we love what we do, our immunity builds automatically.

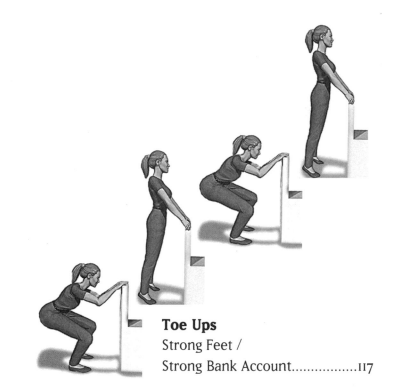

Toe Ups
Strong Feet /
Strong Bank Account.................117

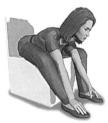

Chin to Shin

Sky Stretch

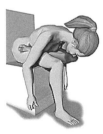

Frog Legs

Face the Feet

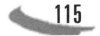

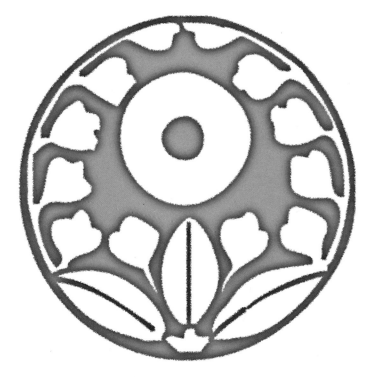

Toe Ups

A 20-second yoga moment

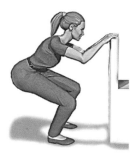

Consider This

Sitting for long hours at a desk or computer can cause your feet and legs to lose their strength and elasticity.

Rationale

"Toe Ups" energizes the lower body, strengthening the hips, legs and feet, and increasing flexibility.

Time to Achieve a Noticeable Result

Two weeks, when done once/day for 20 seconds.

Added Perk

As you strengthen your lower body, it is easier to take the next steps—physically and psychologically.

How To Do "Toe Ups"

- Take off your shoes and hold on to a piece of heavy furniture or a windowsill. Your feet are hip-width apart. Your gaze is parallel to the floor and soft, creating a cocoon of peace around yourself.

- Wiggle your toes and stretch your feet, widening and lengthening them and making a larger footprint on the floor. Exhale; squat and spread your toes. If your knees are weak or previously injured, squat only an inch or two at first.

- Inhale; stand up with your heels lifted. Exhale; stretch up your arches. ☉ Activate your perineum-umbilical lock.

- Inhale; slowly lower your heels while keeping your consciousness raised—toggling on a subtle-energy level between the office environment outside you and the private environment inside you.

- Though your footprint may be small—compared to mountains and corporations—it carries all the power of your presence and the projection of your greatest potential.

In Brief

◈ Soft shoes or no shoes.

◈ Squat.

◈ Stand and lift your heels.

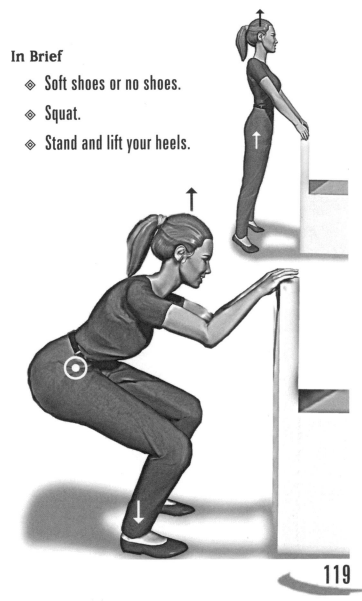

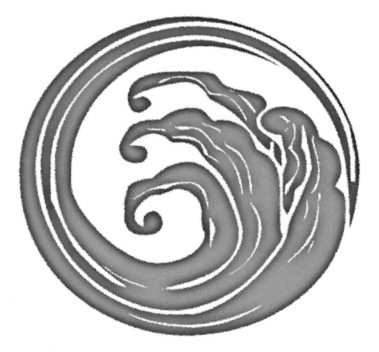

Chin to Shin

A 30-second office yoga moment

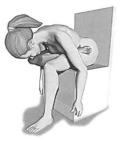

Consider This

Working all day seated at a desk can cause digestion to become sluggish.

Rationale

"Chin to Shin" massages the digestive organs, thus reducing gas after eating, and relieving constipation and the stagnant thoughts that accompany it.

Time to Achieve a Noticeable Result

Three weeks, when done once/day for 30 seconds.

Added Perk

Develops inner conviction to " go with the flow."

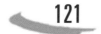

121

How To Do "Chin to Shin"

- Remove your shoes. Push your chair back from your desk. Your left leg is parallel to the chair leg. Your left footprint is firmly placed on the floor with equal pressure front and back and side to side.

- Place the heel of your right foot on top of your left thigh. Optional: it is totally appropriate to modify, so if you have tight hips, place your right foot anywhere in the general vicinity of your left thigh.

- ⊙ Inhale; activate your perineum-umbilical lock. Exhale; squeeze your knees together.

- Breathe naturally and deeply and stretch forward towards the floor. As you come forward, lengthen your spine keeping it straight, rather than rounded. Hold onto the chair legs to pull your head down; or lean on your desk for support and rest your head on your arms. Close your eyes for a moment and relax—inhaling deeply, exhaling fully.

- The next time you do "Chin to Shin" place the heel of your left foot on top of your right thigh. This will help to balance the right and left hemispheres of the brain while strengthening both sides of the body.

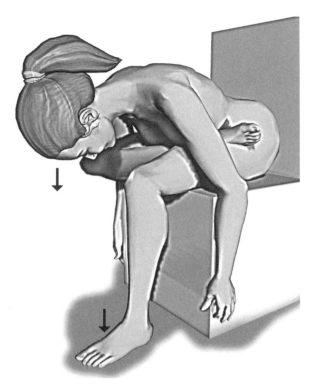

In Brief

◈ Right foot on left thigh.

◈ Squeeze knees together.

◈ Hold chair legs.

◈ Pull head down.

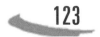

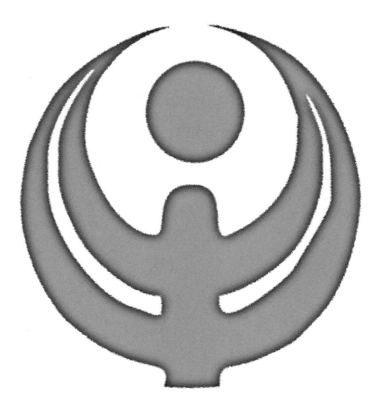

Sky Stretch

A 15-second yoga moment

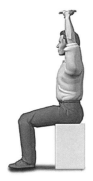

Consider This

Sitting for long hours can cause the spine to compress; diminishing blood flow to the brain and vital organs.

Rationale

"Sky Stretch" helps to increase blood flow the vertebrae, the brain, the lungs, and the digestive organs.

Time to Achieve a Noticeable Result

One week, when done three times/week for 15 seconds.

Added Perk

a) Physical: narrows the waistline. b) Subtle: stretching the guts helps to improve the sense of "right timing."

How To Do "Sky Stretch"

- Sit with your feet hip-width apart. The heels of your feet are under the backs of your knees. Wiggle your toes and broaden your footprints.

- ☉ Inhale; activate your perineum-umbilical lock. Exhale; interlace your fingers, palms up, and reach up.

- Inhale deeply and exhale fully feeling your lungs expand equally on both sides. Lift your chest and your neck as if you feel a puppet string attached to the crown of your head.

- On each inhalation, feel your lungs expand. On each exhalation; reach up, stretching your underarms and lengthening the space between the vertebrae.

- Gaze softly—imagining you can see through the walls of your office and/or through the barriers of your own mind.

- The next time you do "Sky Stretch" change the interlace on your fingers so the other thumb is on top. This will help to balance the right and left hemispheres of the brain while strengthening both sides of the body.

126

In Brief

◈ Interlace fingers; palms up.

◈ Lengthen your neck.

◈ Lift your arms.

◈ Soften your gaze.

◈ Breathe deeply and evenly.

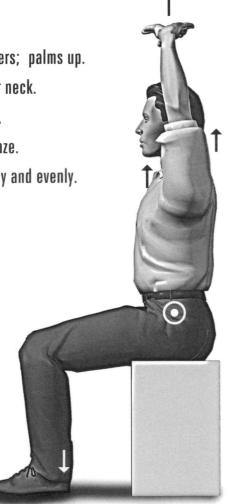

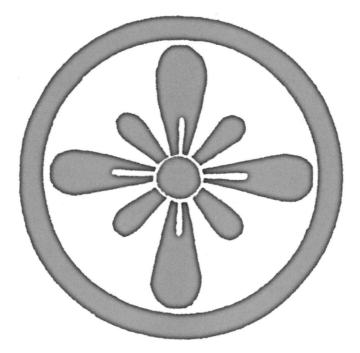

Frog Legs

A 20-second yoga moment

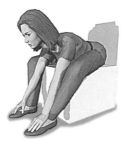

Consider This

Holding the body in tension while working at a computer can lead to rigidity along the spine and a condition of lethargy and a tendency towards procrastination.

Rationale

Frogs look sedentary and lumpy, but they sure can leap. Be poised for action, not stuck in the muck.

Time to Achieve a Noticeable Result

One month, when done two times/week for 20 seconds.

Added Perk

"Frogs Legs" oxygenates the brain; a well-aired brain generates ideas—and makes life more fun.

How To Do "Frog Legs"

- Move your chair back from your desk. Open your knees wide.

- Wiggle your toes one at a time, then stretch your feet, widening and lengthening them and making a larger footprint on the floor. Relax your feet but maintain equal pressure on the arch side and outside of each foot throughout this exercise.

- ⊙ Inhale; activate your perineum-umbilical lock. Exhale; push your buttocks backwards and slide your hands down your shins until your belly is parallel to the floor. Rest your hands on top of your feet. Your chest muscles are firm, your elbows are straight, and your back is as straight as possible.

- Inhale deeply. On each exhalation, stretch your neck forward in line with your spine.

- Soften your gaze or close your eyes. When you feel like it, return your body to its upright position.

Excuse to Boss

"I'm checking the structural integrity of my desk."

In Brief

- ◈ Knees hip-width apart.
- ◈ Slide hands to insteps.
- ◈ Stretch head forward.

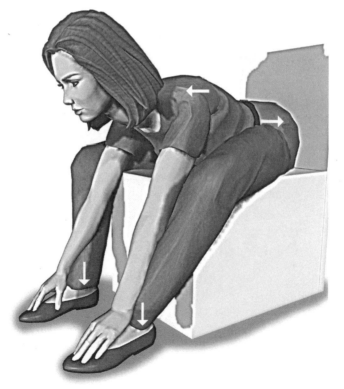

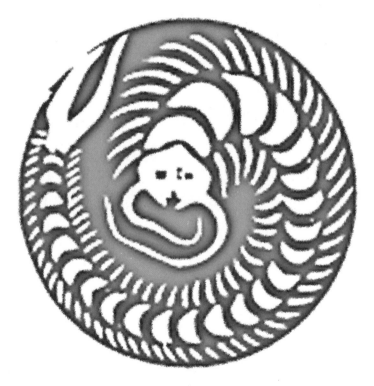

Face the Feet

A 30-second yoga moment

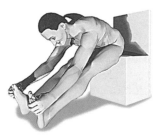

Consider This

We are bombarded every day with stress that can potentially make potholes in our immune systems while simultaneously society nudges us to look younger.

Rationale

"Face the Feet" assists you to achieve a youthful demeanor by increasing your flexibility and strengthening the immune system.

Time to Achieve a Noticeable Result

Two weeks, when done two times/week for 30 seconds.

Added Perk

Flexibility is to the body what compassion is to the mind—worth stretching towards.

How To Do "Face the Feet"

- It's best to do "Face the Feet" in a chair that does not have wheels and when the floor is not slippery.

- Remove your shoes. Scooch back your chair. With straight legs, flex your feet back.

- ⊙ Initiate the perineum-umbilical lock. This will help to protect your low back if your hamstrings are tight. In any case, be careful not to over-stretch your low back; focus more on stretching your chest towards your toes while lengthening your neck.

- Hold the backs of your feet or wherever you can—knees, thighs, or the edge of your desk. Inhale deeply and exhale fully.

- Feel free to squirm, breathing evenly while stretching your breastbone towards your feet and lengthening your neck.

- Soften your gaze or close your eyes. Let your mind share the humility of your feet.

Excuse to Boss

"My mind is sharing the humility of my feet."

134

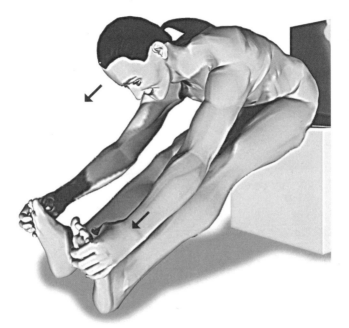

In Brief

- ◈ Remove your shoes.
- ◈ Flex your feet back.
- ◈ Stretch your chest towards your toes.
- ◈ Soften your gaze or close your eyes.

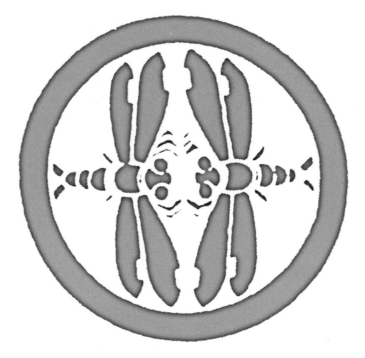

A Yoga Adventure

The principles of yoga—such as breathing *through* a stressful situation and stretching *into* a new level of self-discovery—are applicable in daily living. Here's a personal example....

It is 1978 and I am a flight attendant working on the very first 747 flight to land in Narita, Japan. Until this day, our airplanes have always landed at Haneda Airport and our crews had layovers in Tokyo. Now, with Tokyo over two and a half hours from the new airport in Narita, we are being put up at the only western-style hotel in that vicinity. Few at the hotel speak English— not even the waiters in the restaurant. I speak only a little Japanese. "Please fasten your seatbelt" and "Would you like a pillow?" are about all I can say in Japanese.

The hotel is situated amid rice paddies. It is springtime and the long green rice sprouts undulate in miles of wind. From my room on the 9th floor I see a rice paddy meandering like an emerald green river. I have an urge to flow along with that river.

I drop off my uniform at the hotel laundry and step outside. The air feels fresh. I quickly become absorbed in the countryside. Water lapping. Carp in the fish pond. Pebble paths clicking as I cover ground. Moist mounds of soft grass. Aromatic pine. Fragrance and sound becoming feelings.

I wander into a tunnel of dewy greenery, ducking beneath a giant spider web suspended across the path like a volleyball net. Further along, I duck again for another giant web. This time I stop to watch. The spider appears to be practicing yoga, a Corpse Pose without moving a muscle. The spider's belly faces me through its web—three parallel gold stripes that look to me exactly like our airline pilots' sleeves.

A dragonfly zigzagging ahead, light as air, enters the trap. Iridescent wings flutter desperately. The spider practices an aggressive Spider Pose. As the dragonfly takes her last breath, I exhale along with her and telepathically wish her "good-bye." It is a profound and gentle moment—everything feels very still and very clear, and then I move on.

Further along the path, a small flatbed truck is parked across the path, completely blocking any space to get by. Four Japanese farmers, wearing black cotton boots with a line of sewn-down stitching between the first and second toes, are shoveling something from the

138

bed of the truck into a gully. The farmers look up from their teamwork with a start.

I am afraid of them. Narita Airport has been a political hotbed for nine years. The farmers, resisting the new airport's inevitable pollution and the despoiling of their ancestral lands, instigated over fifty riots. 8,001 people were reportedly injured. After the farmers broke into the newly constructed airport tower and trashed the radar system, the police took control of the airport with tear gas. The radar was repaired and today we are the first commercial jet to land at Narita Airport.

If these farmers ravaged the airport radar, what will they do with me? There are four of them. The path behind me suddenly seems narrow, dark, and full of spider webs. My gut feeling pushes me forward. But the truck blocks me. It is parked across the path leaving no room to pass; not on the engine side, not around the tailgate.

Unless—with a full deep breath and without missing a step—I do a dynamic version of Warrior Pose right through the cab of the truck. I open the door to the cab, slide across the seat and exit through the other door on the driver's side, all in one continuous fluid movement.

139

My maneuver is successful. As I disappear down a bend into the woods, I feel the farmer's eyes boring into my back. Years of flying have left me sensitive to people beckoning for my attention from behind.

I explore the rice paddies for a while, but I don't find any other egress, and I fear it will get dark and I'll be stuck in the paddies overnight.

Suddenly, I feel weak, my knees shaking from hypoglycemia. *I must go back and get some food. I should have brought some fruit, at least.*

Hurriedly, I retrace my steps until I come upon the truck. The farmers are apparently expecting me because the truck is now re-parked parallel to the road with just enough room for me to get by on the right side.

The four farmers are seated cross-legged in the open truck bed with a large thermos and many tiny portions of different foods spread out picnic-style in their midst.

It looks like I can just get by in the narrow space between the truck and the thick forest growth, but I will have to pass within inches of one man.

Just as I approach the truck, that man turns his body in my direction and his muscular arm shoots out towards me. I clearly see his taut bicep and I feel a surge

140

of adrenaline in my gut.

In the split second it takes to complete the last step towards him, I see an orange flash. He has deposited an orange something on the sidegate.

Indeed, it is an orange—the answer to my craving for fruit. I gobble up the orange like a food processor to stop my knees from shaking, peeling it only partially in my haste for a taste, grateful it is an orange and not a fire bomb. The four farmers watch me in silence.

As I finish devouring the fruit, another orange is placed for me on the sidegate. *They are treating me like a wild animal, and I would like to eat another orange.* It is delicious.

This time, however, less hypoglycemic, I peel and savor it, a segment at a time. Simultaneously, I plot my escape, planning ahead as a flight attendant will do. I dare not wait around to find out what they intend to do with their new, blue-eyed pet.

Just as I finish the very last section of the second orange, a pretty box of candy materializes on the sidegate right in front of me. I don't like Japanese candies, their brightly-dyed colors turn me off, and I don't know how to explain this to them.

So, instead, I offer the farmers an explanation

141

for my presence in their woods by demonstrating the full range of my Japanese vocabulary. First, I pronounce the Japanese word for orange, "orang-a," while sucking in some air out of one corner of my mouth, in the Japanese fashion, "Hhssshhhh."

They laugh.

Then I say, in Japanese, "Please fasten your seatbelt," followed by, "Would you like a pillow?"

The farmers giggle, nod, and *ah-so* to each other with every new phrase.

Then, I say "Sayonara." This triggers a heated discussion during which time I become increasingly nervous and antsy to leave. Of course, the discussion is in Japanese and I have no idea what they are saying, but I know it is about me.

Finally, the farmers emerge from their huddle. The one closest to me presents me with another gift. It is a mesh grocery bag with another orange and a packet of miso soup. The soup packet includes a card of a famous Japanese painting from the series, "Views of Mt. Fuji." The painting depicts, in the foreground, a traveler with a knapsack, and, of course, Mt. Fuji in the background. My breathing returns to normal as I realize this is a "going away" present.

I say "thank you" in Japanese and do a modified Homage posture—bowing so low that the crown of my head faces them. My hands are joined in prayer over my heart. This is a very vulnerable posture because you can't see the people you are bowing to. Indeed, I feel vulnerable. But, more than anything, I feel awestruck—that we have managed to vault the *sound* barrier.

I sling the mesh bag over my shoulder and take a deep breath. A thought-form of the "Views of Mt. Fuji" lingers in my mind and I mimic the carriage of the traveler in the painting—bearing his possessions alongside a mountain of hope and dreams.

———

Update: Narita International Airport still retains its barbed-wire police barricades. Meanwhile, every day 67,000 passengers arrive on 170 flights from 38 countries. I wonder how few know the charming adventures that await their discovery if they would but explore just a little.

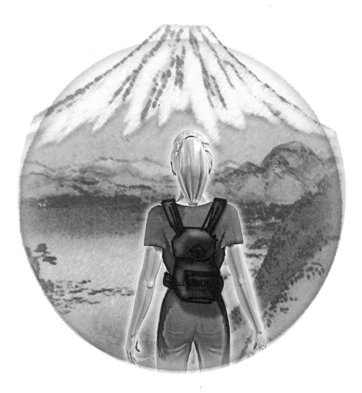

Office Yoga Quiz

1. What is yoga?

    A. The yellow part of an egga.

    B. "Union with God" in Sanskrit.

    C. The way to become a human pretzel.

Answer to I.

A could be true—depending on your dialect. **B** is the correct answer and you will understand this more deeply when you achieve the "Bliss Mist." **C** could also be true—depending on your persistence.

2. If you activate your perineum-umbilical lock (p.29) you will:

    A. Starve.

    B. Find a billfold connected to a cosmic bank account.

    C. Have greater lung capacity.

Answer to 2.

A is false—you certainly won't starve, but you WILL look leaner. **B** is esoterically correct—yoga does create an energetic connection to our divine inheritance. **C** is another correct answer.

3. You are in a "Bliss Mist" (p.25) while in the "Alarm Neutralizer" (p.87) exercise. Suddenly the fire alarm in the building goes off. What should you do?

A. Ignore it. Your bliss is more important than the drill.

B. Activate your perineum-umbilical lock on the source of the flames.

C. Find an exit and get out.

Answer to 3.

A or **C** are correct. As to whether you should ignore the fire alarm or exit the building immediately, you need to follow your own gut feelings. No one can tell you how to live your life. **B** is intruiging; if you know how to activate your-perineum-umbilical lock *on the source* of the flames, please contact me. I want to learn this esoteric practice.

146

4. When your boss catches you doing "Homage," you should say:

> A. I'm begging for a raise.
> B. I'm envisioning the rise in profits that will come from taking better care of myself.
> C. I beg your pardon.

Answer to 4.

Whatever will keep you employed is certainly the correct response. Office Yoga is not about being a drop out.

5. You're faced with doing four hours of audio transcription, so what are the best postures to prepare for this?

> A. "Rump? What Rump?"
>   "Homage"
>   "Hump? What Hump?"
> B. "Toe Ups"
>   "Hump? What Hump?"
>   "Pin Ups"
> C. "Hump? What Hump?"
>   "Toe Ups"
>   "Thyroid Thrill"

Answer to 5.

The rigid form and repetitive, but constrained hand and foot movements that accompany transcription work are best served by the postures listed in Answer C. "Hump? What Hump?," "Toe Ups," and "Thyroid Thrill."

6. What is a yogi?

A. A close companion of a Boo-Boo.

B. An adult who wears a diaper.

C. A person who senses undercurrents and penetrates subtle energies.

The rest of the answers to the "Office Yoga Quiz" can be found on the Web at www.flyana.com/yogaquiz.html. Alternately, please send a self-addressed, stamped envelope with one dollar, and you will receive the rest of the answers by snail mail.

---

7. Guess how many OFFICE YOGA exercises are named after animals?

A. 2—Swan and frog.

B. 1—Spider.

C. 3—Rat, dragonfly, and cockroach.

148

8. Which OFFICE YOGA exercise could be mistaken for provocative body language?

    A. "Alarm Neutralizer" (p.87).

    B. "Hump? What Hump?" (p.57).

    C. "Thyroid Thrill" (p.99).

9. What is the meaning of the term "Monolith of Mastery"?

    A. A nickname for the home of Bill Gates.

    B. An exercise to help gain physical balance.

    C. A phrase that when said with a deep booming voice impresses women and frightens small children.

10. Which OFFICE YOGA exercise (if you do it with your eyes open) will run you the risk of being given time off for mental health reasons?

    A. All of them.

    B. "Focus Time" (p.107).

    C. Spider.

11. Which causes carpal tunnel syndrome?

    A. Typing.

    B. Pushing an airline beverage cart at 30,000 feet.

    C. Burrowing in the sand for water.

12. What is Sanskrit?

    A. Writing with a stick on a sandy beach.

    B. A woman's skirt worn only to the beach.

    C. An ancient language from India.

13. Which items on your desktop could injure you when you do OFFICE YOGA?

    A. The joystick for your video games.

    B. Your automatic stapler.

    C. Matches.

14. Which body parts may end up on your desktop—all at the same time—when you do OFFICE YOGA?

    A. Elbows, perineum, thyroid.

    B. Achilles, palms, crown.

    C. Aura, palms, fingertips.

15. When you are performing the "Swan Stretch" (p.61), if you can't get your first arm behind you, what should you do next?

    A. Ask a co-worker to try a half-Nelson.

    B. Try anyway. It's the effort that counts—not the achievement.

    C. Skip it and do a swan dive.

16. What is a "perineum" (p.29)?

    A. A close relative of a periwinkle.

    B. When strengthened, it will put "adult diapers" out of business.

    C. The Roman god of aqueducts.

17. What is "fuzzy focus" (p.22)?

    A. An hallucination.

    B. A childhood toy.

    C. A way to improve your eyesight.

18. What is the origin of "Telecom Twist"?

    A. Changing long distance carriers often.

    B. Not needing rollers on your office chair.

    C. A merger between the telephone company and the Communist Party.

19. What do you tell a colleague who wants to take your OFFICE YOGA to the copy machine?

    A. It has a copyright protected by a Sanskrit curse.

    B. Diana's a friend of mine and she'd really be upset if I let you do that.

    C. You look like you need your own copy.

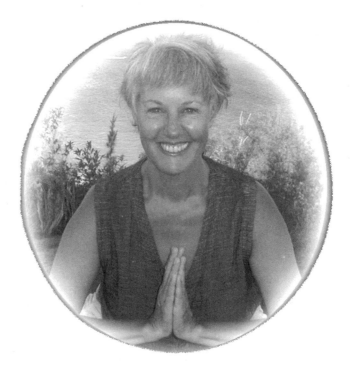

About the Author

During my college years, I spent ten months in Paris studying French—literature, art, history, even cooking.

One evening, coming out of the *metro* (subway) near my *residence* on the Left Bank, I saw a flyer posted on a wall. It said, "yoga" with an address scribbled in pencil.

All night I was obsessively intrigued with the idea of studying yoga, and the next day I found the flyer again and copied down the address. Then, after my classes, I found this address—an apartment on the Right Bank.

The door was open. Sitting on a Persian rug was the first yogi I'd ever seen.

He was naked except for a white loincloth. I remember wondering, *Why isn't this skinny guy cold,* and then, *Am I safe? Is he a nut?*

Yes. Yes. I was safe. He wasn't a nut. He was a

Spaniard who spoke almost no French and absolutely no English. I was struggling in French and spoke no Spanish. But this turned out to be good for me—because the unusual circumstances quieted my mind. The yogi couldn't answer my questions, so my mind stopped questioning. Instead, I'd return every day and copied—without much difficulty—all the postures he demonstrated. The Lotus. The Head Stand. It all seemed so natural and so much fun.

There, on a beautiful old Persian rug on the Right Bank, I re-discovered my love for yoga. I say "re-discovered" because I believe I've lived before and done yoga before.

This pattern of re-discovering yoga then repeated itself again and again during this current incarnation—because I had lacked the discipline to persist in my practice of yoga.

Foolishly, I'd forget yoga for years—only to come back to it again—needy, tired and injured.

During my twenty-one years as an international flight attendant, I had two major injuries and both nearly killed me.

During my first year of flying, I had a pulmonary embolism. I was climbing the mechanics' stairway to the aircraft in spike heels, my hands full of aircraft supplies, when the aluminum door swung back in a gust of wind and hit my leg, bruising the calf.

During two long flights in pressurized aircraft from the West Coast to Tokyo and back, the leg swelled up to more than twice normal size. The night I got home, I woke up with a severe pain in my chest. A blood clot had passed through my heart and lodged in my right lung.

At the hospital, I had to stretch the lung open by breathing pressurized air. Sucking pressurized air is not painful—but it is definitely at the edge of pain. My comfort zone became broader through this therapy, and I now enjoy a similar sensation while ballooning my lungs when I practice yoga. It makes me happy. Maybe that's due to the intense sensation of expanding my lungs, which brings me right to the edge of my mortality—the thin thread that offers me life with every breath.

The second injury came two decades later—this time caused by poisons in my workplace, toxic air that recirculates in commercial jet cabins. This injury ended my flying career.

The toxicity in airplane air is a combination of jet fuel, hydraulic fluid leaks, engine lubricant oil, cleaning compounds, and pesticides that are sprayed on passengers and crew as a landing requirement in many countries. (My book JET SMARTER presents readers with the many environmental hazards of air travel and offers over 200 tips on how to beat the system and beat jetlag.)

The chemical injury I suffered while flying is something I still live with today, more than a decade after being "medically grounded." Toxic chemicals affect me—even structurally. I'll explain. Toxins affect the immune system, as most people know. But what I also experience is that my ability to hold myself erect—my structure—is affected by toxins. In other words, my back can "go out" in the presence of even small amounts of poisonous chemical vapors.

People who have been systemically poisoned experience recurring injuries from everyday toxins. Even so-called "normal" doses of poison (like driving behind a diesel truck or sleeping in a room with a new carpet) are interpreted by my body as assaults. My doctor, George Ewing, M.D., explains: "Chemical exposures work on your nervous system—and your nervous system is hooked up to all your muscles. This is why your back is influenced by your chemical sensitivity."

So, today, for me, these recurring back injuries make yoga a vital source of recovery—just to be functional. Life has required me to find a way to set myself straight. This is the origin of OFFICE YOGA.

Books, Consulting, Speaking

OFFICE YOGA: At-Your-Desk Exercises

A series of yoga exercises for computer workers developed by Diana as her own therapeutic practice.

OFFICE YOGA, autographed, $9.95
Shipping/Handling, $4.50 U.S./$10 international

NONI: Aspirin of the Ancients

Noni is an herb used as a traditional remedy for cancer, high blood pressure, arthritis, worms and diabetes. A veteran international flight attendant, Diana became severely ill from routine spraying of pesticides in aircraft cabins; then she took noni to detoxify.

"NONI is a decidedly enchanting book of fact and herbal wisdom with a friendly folklore feel to it. This is another fine example of Fairechild's wonderful talent. She naturally and easily captures in her writing a mystical lightness that connects us to our better selves, that brings us closer to our creator—all in the context of solid, usable, unique information."

—Linda A. Evans, Atlanta Wellness Journal

NONI, Autographed $9.95
Shipping/Handling, $4.50 U.S./$10 international

JET SMARTER: The Air Traveler's Rx

There are dangers in air travel, some obvious, many hidden. The air in commercial jets is toxic. And the oxygen is inadequate—pilots get ten times more fresh air than passengers. Pesticides are sprayed on seats, on luggage, and sometimes right on passengers. Radiation for frequent flyers equals that of atomic energy workers. Drawing on 21 years' experience as an airline insider, Fairechild gives readers a rare, no-holds-barred look at the dangers of air travel and offers hundreds of sensible ways to cope with or even avoid their impact on one's health. JET SMARTER can startle readers with how hazardous airline practices are, comfort readers with the author's personally-tested approach to surviving the air travel experience, and entertain readers with Diana Fairechild's sometimes gentle, sometimes gritty, but always grand sense of humor.

"Fairechild discusses all the health hazards endemic to airline travel."—Andrew Weil, M.D.

"A hot-selling treatise on jetlag."—Forbes

JET SMARTER, autographed, $14.95
Shipping/Handling $4.50 U.S./$10 international

THE FAIR AIR COALITION

The Fair Air Coalition, founded by Fairechild in 1997, is a tax-exempt, nonprofit advocacy group run by airline passengers. Activities include focusing media attention on aviation health as an issue of air travel safety and educating the flying public on flight-induced maladies. To become a member of the Fair Air Coalition, make a donation in any amount. Call (808) 828-1919 to donate by MasterCard, Visa or Amex.

"Fairechild is a consumer rights activist."—TIME Magazine

SPEAKING

Diana Fairechild teaches seminars to groups and corporations on minimizing the ill effects of jet travel and maximizing productivity and efficiency after flying. She also speaks on the subjects of detoxification, office yoga, fear of flying, and self publishing. Fairechild has been quoted by *Forbes, Smart Money, USA Today, Conde Nast Traveler, The National Law Journal, Whole Earth Review* and CNN. She is the author of four books and has written freelance for ABCNews.com and Reuters News Service. Prior to writing and speaking, she served as an international flight attendant for 21 years, flying 10 million miles around the world. Arrange for Diana Fairechild to speak to your group anywhere in the world. Her enthusiasm is inspiring. For easy to follow, engaging presentations, call 808/828-1919.

"It is magical to see so many writers, all with different projects at different levels of doneness, and watch their books come to fruition in Diana's course. The classes are interactive, so they take on a life of their own."—J. VanPelt, Executive, Kauai Electric

For More Information

Publisher: Flyana Rhyme Publishing
Tel / Fax: 808 828-1919
WWW: www.flyana.com
Email: diana@flyana.com
Post: PO Box 248
Anahola, Hawaii 96703-USA

Consulting

Speaking

Books